THE PROGRAM

Eat It Lift It Love It

NO EXCUSES

By Ashley and Stephen Ross

DEDICATION

This book is dedicated to our beautiful daughter, Bailey. We only hope to be good role models and give you the tools to live a healthy and happy life. We Love You.

Ashley E Ross

Eat it. Lift it. Love it. No Excuses!

CONTENTS

Eat it. Lift it. Love it. No Excuses!

THE BASIC RULES OF THE PROGRAM

1. Rid your cupboards of cheat foods.
2. Be Prepared. Plan and Cook your meals the day before.
3. Get cheap tupperware (8-10 containers). You will need them to prep the next days meals.
4. Eat 5-6 meals per day. For Example 7am, 10am, 1pm, 4pm, 7pm.
5. Try to eat your last meal of the day at least 2 hours before bed.
6. Satisfy your sweet cravings with a protein bar or shake.
7. Eat the majority of your carbohydrates during meals #2-4.
8. Allow yourself 1 cheat meal per week.
9. Drink water and only water. Preferably 3-4 liters per day.
10. Multivitamins are good. We also suggest fish oil and glucosamine for joint health.
11. Eat within 30 minutes of a workout, preferable a whey protein shake and banana. We recommend a lean whey protein, at this time we use Dymatize Nutrition Elite All Natural Whey Protein.
12. No sugary add ons. Instead spice up your meals with salsa, hot sauce, Mrs Dash seasoning and cinnamon.
13. To save money- buy in bulk. You are going to use it. We shop for the majority of our food at Costco.

To maximize weight loss results.

Calculate your dietary needs. In order to figure out what your daily intake should be, use the following formula using your ideal body weight (IBW):

$((IBW \times 10) \times 1.6) - 500 =$ Daily calories

These values are based on the recommended 5 days per week of exercise at 30-45 minutes per day. Once you have calculated the number of calories you should eat per day, you can then calculate the number of grams of carbohydrates, proteins and fats. We recommend an intake of 30% Protein, 30% Fats, 40% Carbs. To calculate these amounts use the following formulas:

Protein: (Daily calories x 0.3)/4= grams of protein/day
Carbs: (Daily calories x 0.4)/4= grams of carbs/day
Fats: (Daily calories x 0.3)/9= grams of fat/day

Example: My ideal body weight is 130lbs.
$((130 \times 10) \times 1.6) - 500 = 1580$ calories/day
$(1580 \times 0.3)/4 = 118.5$g protein/day
$(1580 \times 0.4)/4 = 158$g carbs/day
$(1580 \times 0.3)/9 = 52$g fat/day

Eat it. Lift it. Love it. No Excuses!

From the Creators

How The Program was created:

THE PROGRAM was originally developed by Stephen Ross after completing his Bachelors degree in Exercise Physiology, Minor in Nutrition and NSCA Personal Trainer Certification. He used the combination of exercise and nutrition to gain effective and lasting results for his clients and himself. Years later we have altered and incorporated it into our present lives. Stephen now works as a Flight Paramedic, on 24 hour shifts, and I, Ashley, as a Nurse, with random hours. Did I mention we also have a toddler. After giving birth to our daughter my body changed drastically. I developed a gluten intolerance and an under active thyroid, which lowered my metabolism. I was not bouncing back into my pre-baby body like everyone said I would. I breastfed for a full year and didn't loose 1 single pound. I needed to make a change. Knowing my husbands background I asked him to train me and to teach me what I needed to do in order to get back into shape. We developed an exercise and nutrition program that would work with our crazy schedule while catering to my new gluten free needs. The results were amazing. In 3 months I was in better shape than I was before I was pregnant. I could see the fronts of my hip bones again, my waistline returned and my butt even started to perk up. From then on we began constantly coaching each other. When we are out of the house with comments like, "Thats not on The Program" people around us eventually started asking questions. What was this program we were on and what were we doing to get these great results? So now we have made it official. This is our life and it is fabulous, we love being in the kitchen together and the gym. I grew up being overweight and have never found anything that worked for me until now. It is the most efficient and healthy way to live and it works for our busy lifestyle.

How Does it work:

The Program works by combining both nutrition and exercise to reach your health and fitness goals. You cannot have one without the other and get lasting results. Yes, you can just diet and not workout but then you are skinny fat and chances are you will get fat again. We believe the body has muscle memory, as well as, fat memory. This is our theory for why crash diets never work. When you do a crash diet you loose fat but also muscle. Your fat cells don't go away they shrink in size. So when you return to your old habits they regrow with a vengeance. This program is designed to burn fat while building muscle. We want to the body to gain muscle and develop new muscle memory to replace the size of the fat cells its used to. By doing this you increase your metabolism and create an athletic, healthy physique we like to call -Fit.

Eat it. Lift it. Love it. No Excuses!

How is this different from other diets:

The program teaches healthy habits that last in order for you to reach your goals, as well as maintain them. It you are looking to get skinny fast, well, good luck and pick up this book when that doesn't workout for you. If you are looking to get a lean, athletic build, well you've come to the right place. This program is nothing new, theres no magic or miracles. This is simply a handbook giving you the tools to live a healthy and happy life. Its up to you to make it happen! No one is going to do it for you.

*Always consult your primary care provider before beginning a new exercise or diet program

Morning Meals

Example 1
>2 **Protein Pancakes** w/ low sugar syrup
>Multi-vitamin, fish oil and glucosamine
>Water

Example 2
>3 egg whites scrambled with 1 whole egg
>1-2 tablespoons Pico de Gallo salsa
>2 corn tortillas
>Multi-vitamin, fish oil and glucosamine
>Water

Example 3
>2 Brown Rice Cakes
>1 **Pumpkin Pie Protein Shake**
>Multi-vitamin, fish oil and glucosamine
>Water

Example 4
>3/4 cup **Power** or **Apple oatmeal**
>Multi-vitamin, fish oil and glucosamine
>Water

Example 5
>2 **Protein Waffles**
>1 handful or 1/2 cup berries on top
>Multi-vitamin, fish oil and glucosamine
>Water

Example 6
>**Sweet Potato Hash**
>4 egg whites scrambled
>Multi-vitamin, fish oil, and glucosamine
>Water

Eat it. Lift it. Love it. No Excuses!

Snacks

Example 1
  1 medium apple
  1/2 tablespoon Cinnamon
  Water

Example 2
  2 Brown Rice Cakes
  2 Tablespoons of all natural Peanut Butter or Almond Butter (no added sugar)
  Water

Example 3
  1 medium Banana or preferred piece of fruit
  Water

Example 4
  1 **Egg Nog Protein Shake**
  Water

Example 5
  1 handful of Raw Almonds
  Water

Example 6
  1/2 cup greek yogurt
  1/2 Apple sliced
  Water

Eat it. Lift it. Love it. No Excuses!

Afternoon Meals

Example 1
    4oz **Turkey Burger**
    5oz yam
    Water

Example 2
    4 oz chicken breast (about the size of deck of cards)
    1/4 cup brown rice
    1 cup broccoli
    Water

Example 3
    1/2 cup LF cottage cheese (try w/cinnamon and a bit of honey)
    1/4 cup crushed pineapple or equivalent
    1/2 cup Edamame
    Water

Example 4
    Spring mix lettuce
    2 oz avocado
    1 tablespoon **Sweet Basil Salad Dressing**
    1/4 cup tomatoes
    1/8 cup onion
    4 oz turkey or chicken breast
    Water

Example 5
    1 cup raw cabbage
    4 oz chicken breast
    2 soft corn tortillas
    2 tablespoon Pico de Gallo Salsa
    Water

Eat it. Lift it. Love it. No Excuses!

Evening Meals

Example 1
>1 serving **Chicken and Shrimp Stir-fry**
>Water

Example 2
>1 serving **Blue Cheese Turkey Muffins**
>5 oz Asparagus
>Water

Example 3
>4 oz Flank Steak
>1 tablespoon **Sweet Basil Dressing**
>1 cup Spring mix lettuce
>1/4 cup tomatoes
>1/8 cup onion
>Water

Example 4
>4 oz chicken breast
>1 cup broccoli
>Water

Example 5
>4 oz Tilapia or Salmon
>1 cup broccoli
>1/4 Avocado
>1 wedge of lemon
>Water

Home Workout

4 days of the following routine, plus and additional 2 days, 30-45 minutes of cardio

50 jumping jacks

20 squats

30 second mountain climbers

30 second planks

10 jump squats

20 standing calf raises

10 lunges (each leg)

50 crunches

5 knee push ups

repeat 3x

Eat it. Lift it. Love it. No Excuses!

Gym Workout

Day 1 Back Biceps Abs

    10 Minute Cardio Warmup

    Seated Cable Row 3sets x 15 reps

    Wide grip pull down 3x15

    Close grip pull down 3x15

    Alternating bicep Curls 3x15

    Bar bell bicep curls 3x15

    Crunches 100-200

    Hanging knee or leg raises

    Planks 1min x 5sets

Day 2 Chest Shoulders Triceps

    10 Minute Cardio Warmup

    Barbell Chest press 3x15

    Push ups 3x10

    Dumbbell Shoulder press 3x 15

    Lateral Raises 3x 15

    Front dumbbell raises 3x 15

    Kneeling dumbbell row 3x15

    Cable press down 3x15

Eat it. Lift it. Love it. No Excuses!

Day 3 Legs/Glutes

10 Minute Cardio Warmup

Lunges 20x4

Knee extension 3x15

Glute cable kickback 3x15 each leg

Hack squats 3x15

Stiff legged dead lifts 3x15

Leg press 3x15

Step ups 25 step ups each leg x   2

Leg curls laying 3x 15

Leg curls seated 3x15

Day 4 Cardio HIIT/spin class preferred

Day 5 Cardio HIIT/spin class preferred

Eat it. Lift it. Love it. No Excuses!

Eat it. Lift it. Love it. No Excuses!

Breakfast

Protein Pancakes
Pumpkin Protein Pancakes
Cornbread Waffles
Protein Waffles
Monkey Protein Shake
Power Oatmeal
French Toast Omelet
Sweet Potato Hash
Apple Oatmeal
Detox Juice
Homemade Protein Bars
Peppermint Protein Shake
Egg Nog Protein Shake
Pumpkin Pie Protein Shake
Peppermint Mocha Protein Shake

Eat it. Lift it. Love it. No Excuses!

Protein Pancakes

Serves 3
1/4 cup Whole Rolled Oats
1/2 cup Fat Free Cottage Cheese
11 Egg Whites
1 Whole Egg
2 tsp Cinnamon
1 tsp Vanilla

Combine all ingredients into blender. Blend until smooth. Pour pancake on non stick skillet over medium heat. Each pancake is approximately 4 inch in diameter. Flip when side down is brown. Done when both sides are brown. Serve immediately.

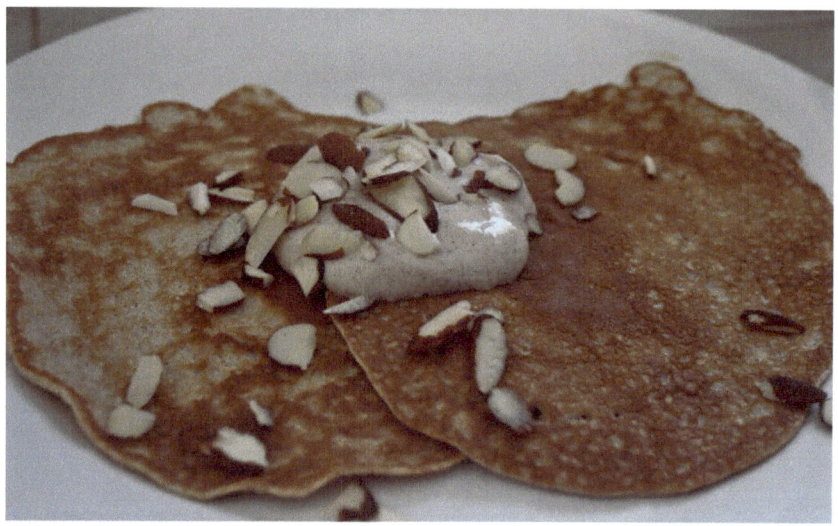

Serving size 2 pancakes
Total Calories 146
Total Fat 0.8 g
Total Carbs 9.2 g
Total Protein 29.6 g
Total Sugar 2.8 g

Eat it. Lift it. Love it. No Excuses!

Pumpkin Protein Pancakes

Serves 3
1/4 cup Whole Rolled Oats
1/2 cup Fat Free Cottage Cheese
1/2 can Pure Pumpkin Puree
11 Egg Whites
1 Whole Egg
2 tsp Pumpkin Pie Seasoning

Combine all ingredients into blender. Blend until smooth. Pour pancake on non stick skillet over medium heat. Each pancake is approximately 4 inch in diameter. Flip when side down is brown. Done when both sides are brown. Serve immediately.

Serving size 2 pancakes
Total Calories 230
Total Fat 2.7 g
Total Carbs 18.5 g
Total Protein 34.7 g
Total Sugar 7.5 g

Cornbread Waffles

Serves 2-3
1 cup Gluten Free Whole Grain Yellow Cornmeal
1 cup Fat Free Cottage Cheese
2 cups liquid egg whites or 12 egg whites

Combine all ingredients into blender. Blend until smooth. Pour into waffle maker and cook until browned. Top with a handful of your favorite berries. Serve immediately.

Serving size 2 Waffles
Total Calories 290
Total Fat 3.2 g
Total Carbs 34.6 g
Total Protein 28 g
Total Sugar 3 g

Eat it. Lift it. Love it. No Excuses!

Protein Waffles

Serves 2-3
1 cup Whole Rolled Oats
1 cup Fat Free Cottage Cheese
2 cups liquid egg whites or 12 egg whites
2 Tbsp ground Flax Seed

Combine all ingredients into blender. Blend until smooth. Pour into waffle maker and cook until   browned. Top with a handful of your favorite berries. Serve immediately.

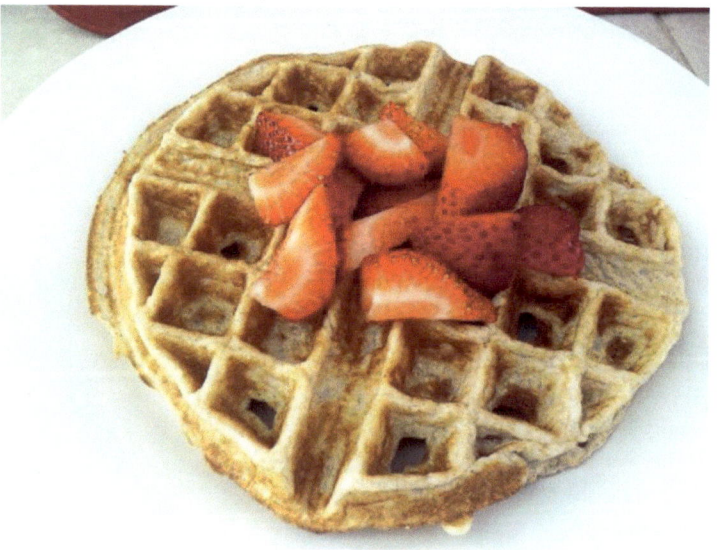

Serving size 2 Waffles
Total Calories 194
Total Fat 2.6 g
Total Carbs 12.4 g
Total Protein 26.4 g
Total Sugar 3 g

Not-So-Chunky Monkey Protein Shake

Serves 1
1 scoop of Chocolate Whey Protein
8 oz Vanilla Almond Milk Unsweetened
1 Tbsp Natural Peanut Butter- no sugar added
1 Banana

Add ingredients listed to blender add ice or not your choice. Blend and enjoy!

Serving size 1 shake
Total Calories 485
Total Fat 14.4 g
Total Carbs 39 g
Total Protein 54.5 g
Total Sugar: 16g

Power Oatmeal

Serves 3
1 cup Whole Rolled Oats
2 cups Water
2 Large Egg Whites
1/4 cup Raisins
1/4 cup Unsalted Dry Roasted Slivered Almonds
1 Tbsp Cinnamon

Bring 2 cups of water to boil in medium sauce pan. Add oatmeal and cook at a simmer. When almost all water is absorbed add raisins, cinnamon, and egg whites. Fold into oatmeal until egg whites turn white and are fully cooked. Add nuts and enjoy.

Serving size 1/3 of Total Mixture
Total Calories 246
Total Fat 7.4 g
Total Carbs 35.5 g
Total Protein 9.1 g
Total Sugar 10.7g

Eat it. Lift it. Love it. No Excuses!

French Toast Omelet

Serves 1
5 Large egg whites
1 tsp Vanilla
1 tspCinnamon
1 spray butter flavored pam cooking spray
1/2 medium banana sliced
1/2 Tbsp Honey

Combine eggs, vanilla, and cinnamon in small bowl. Mix well. In medium skillet or omelet pan, spray with butter pam cooking spray and add   mixture over medium heat. While edges of egg mixture are firm on the bottom but still a little runny on top, sprinkle in banana slices. Use your spatula to gently lift around the edges of the omelette to make sure it is not sticking. Gently roll the sides of your omelette, slowly folding the ends of the omelet, closing in the banana. Roll Omelette onto your spatula and transfer to plate. drizzle with honey and enjoy!

Serving size 1 Omelette
Total Calories 186
Total Fat 0.4g
Total Carbs 27.4 g
Total Protein 20.9 g
Total Sugar 15.4

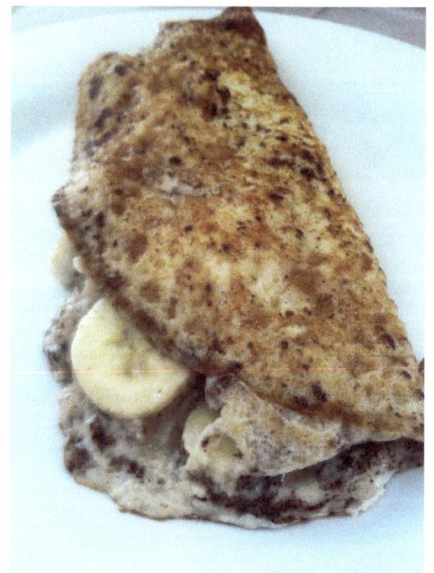

Sweet Potato Hash

Serves 6
3 large Yams peeled and cubed
1 chopped bell pepper orange
1 medium shallot chopped
2 stalks green onion chopped
1/2 Tbsp coconut oil
1/4 tsp Garlic salt
1/4 tsp Perfect Pinch Salt free fiesta lime
1/4 tsp Onion powder
pinch of Pepper

Heat coconut oil in large pan on medium high heat. Add all ingredients when heated and mix well. Cover and cook approximately 20 min stirring occasionally or until sweet potato is al dente or to preferred texture. For the egg, I combine 4 egg whites and 1 whole egg in a measuring cup. And pour together in a pan, cook like a fried egg. It's great on top of the hash and gets your protein in!

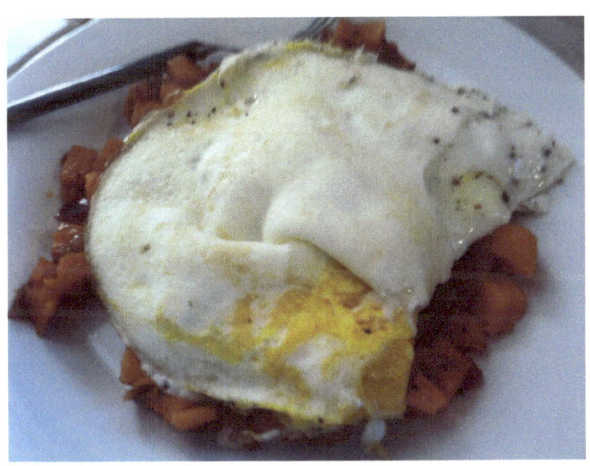

Serving size 1/6 of dish
Total Calories 277
Total Fat 2.5 g
Total Carbs 42.8g
Total Protein 2.2g
Total Sugar 0.9g

Eat it. Lift it. Love it. No Excuses!

Apple Oatmeal

Serves 3
1 cup Whole Rolled Oats
2 cups Water
2 large Egg Whites
1 small Fuji Apple Cubed
1 Tbsp Cinnamon

Bring 2 cups of water to boil in medium sauce pan. Add oatmeal and cook at a simmer. When almost all water is absorbed add apples, cinnamon, and egg whites. Fold into oatmeal until egg whites turn white and are fully cooked.

Serving size 1/3 of Total Mixture
Total Calories 165
Total Fat 2.4g
Total Carbs 28.8g
Total Sugar 5g
Total Protein 7.4g

Detox Juice

Serves 8
6 Fuji Apples
5 Medium Navel Oranges
5 cups Raw Baby Spinach
3 large Carrots
5 slices Ginger Root

Juice and combine all ingredient.

Serving size 1 cup
Total Calories 89
Total Fat 0.1g
Total Carbs 31.5g
Total Protein 1.3g
Total Sugar 21.8g

Eat it. Lift it. Love it. No Excuses!

Homemade Protein Bars

Serves 8
2 cups Quick Oats
1 cup Chocolate Whey Protein
1/4 cup Raisins
1 Tbsp Cinnamon
1 Tbsp Vanilla
1/4 cup Peanut Butter
1/4 90% Cocoa Chocolate Baking Bar
1/4 cup Applesauce (no sugar added)
1/4 cup slivered Almonds
2 Tbsp Extra Virgin Coconut Oil

Mix all dry ingredient in large bowl. In separate medium bowl, mix all wet ingredients including chocolate and microwave for 30 seconds. Stir. Then add wet ingredients to dry ingredients and combine. Place parchment paper in 8x8 baking sheet and pour in batter. Smooth until even and refrigerate for 20 min. Cut into 8 equal parts. Store in fridge.

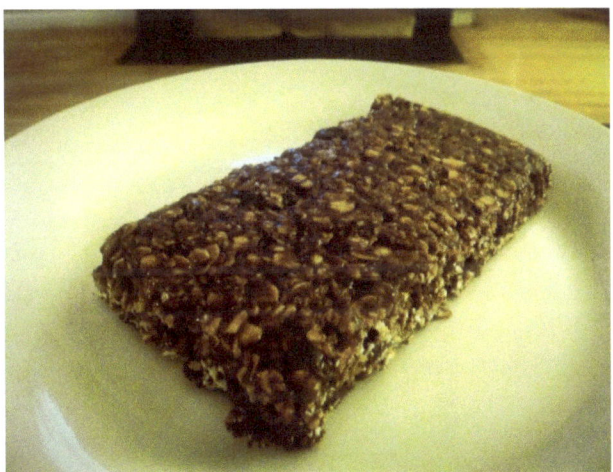

Serving size 1 Bar
Total Calories 282
Total Fat 14.6g
Total Carbs 23.9g
Total Protein 17g
Total Sugar 5g

Eat it. Lift it. Love it. No Excuses!

Peppermint Protein Shake

Serves 1
1 cup Silk Almond Milk Original
6 ice cubes
1.5 scoops All Natural Vanilla Whey Protein
1/4 tsp Peppermint extract
1 packet Stevia Sweetener

Mix all ingredients in the blender. Blend and Enjoy!

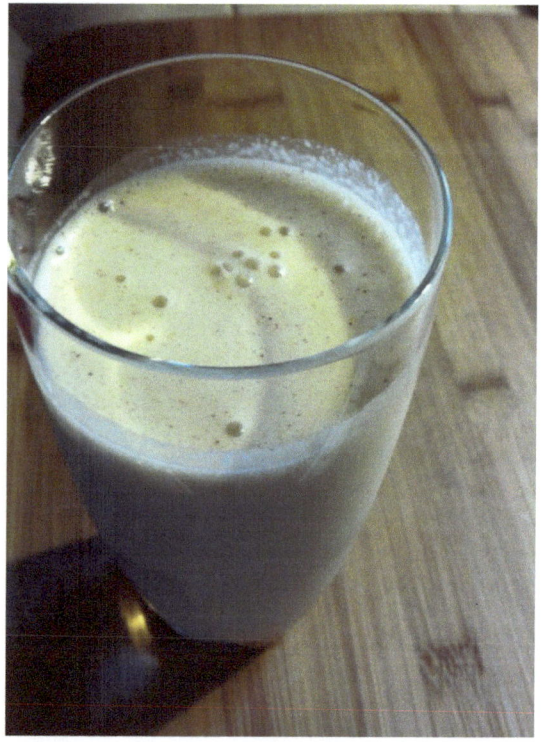

Serving size 1 Shake
Total Calories 282
Total Fat 14.6g
Total Carbs 23.9g
Total Protein 17g
Total Sugar 5g

Eat it. Lift it. Love it. No Excuses!

Egg Nog Protein Shake

Serves 1
1 cup Silk Almond Milk Original
6 ice cubes
1.5 scoops All Natural Vanilla Whey Protein
1/4 tsp ground nutmeg
1/2 tsp ground cinnamon
1/4 tsp ground ginger
1 dash Ground Cloves
1/2 tsp Vanilla Extract Gluten Free
1 packet Stevia Sweetener

Mix all ingredients in the blender. Blend and   Enjoy

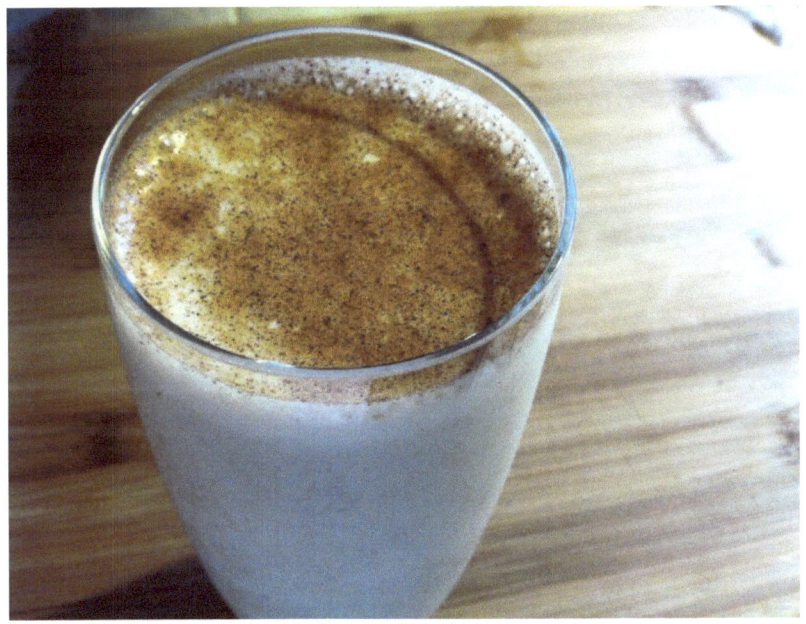

Serving size 1 shake
Total Calories 229
Total Fat 5.8g
Total Carbs 8.7g
Total Protein 37.1g
Total Sugar 0.2g

Eat it. Lift it. Love it. No Excuses!

Pumpkin Pie Protein Shake

Serves 1
1 cup Silk Almond Milk Original
6 ice cubes
1/2 cup Pumpkin Puree
1.5 scoops All Natural Vanilla Whey Protein
1/2 tsp Pumpkin Pie Spice
1/2 tsp ground cinnamon
1/2 tsp Vanilla Extract Gluten Free
1 packet Stevia Sweetener

Mix all ingredients in the blender. Blend and Enjoy!

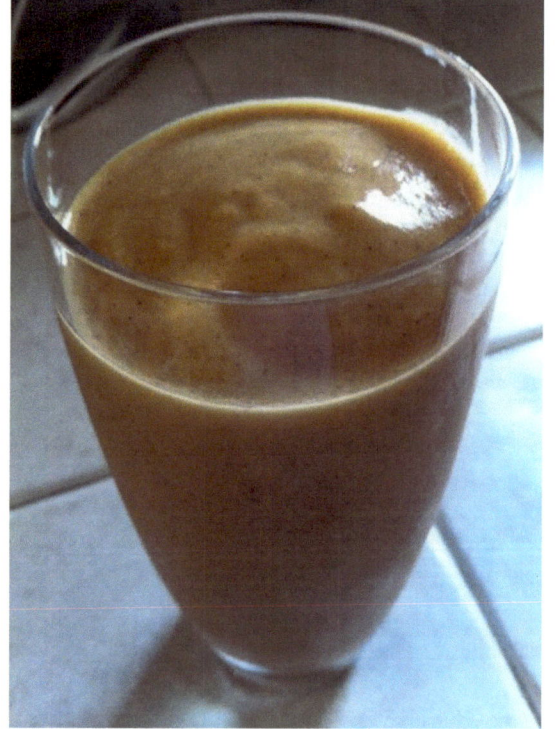

Serving size 1 Shake
Total Calories 264
Total Fat 6g
Total Carbs 16.8g
Total Protein 39g
Total Sugar 4g

Eat it. Lift it. Love it. No Excuses!

Peppermint Mocha Protein Shake

Serves 1
1 cup Silk Almond Milk Original
6 ice cubes
1.5 scoops All Natural Chocolate Whey Protein
1Tbsp All Natural Peanut Butter
1/2 tbsp Unsweetened Cocoa Powder
1 packet Stevia Sweetener
1/8 tsp Peppermint Flavoring

Mix all ingredients in the blender. Blend and Enjoy!

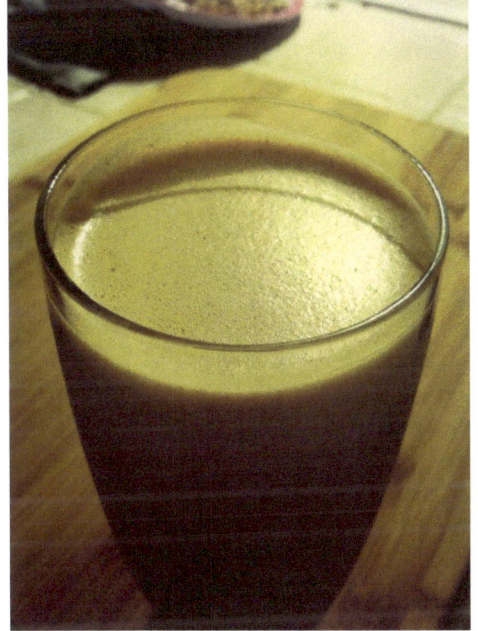

Serving size 1 Shake
Total Calories 216
Total Fat 6g
Total Carbs 7g
Total Protein 38g
Total Sugar 0g

Eat it. Lift it. Love it. No Excuses!

Eat it. Lift it. Love it. No Excuses!

Sides

Baked Caramelized Yam
Mashed Sweet Potato
Sweet Potato Fries
Sweet Basil Dressing
Oven Roasted Vegetable Medley
Asian Coleslaw

Eat it. Lift it. Love it. No Excuses!

Caramelized Yams

Serves 6
3 medium yams
Butter flavored Pam cooking spray
Dash of Salt

Cut sweet potato into 1/2 - 3/4in slices. Place slices on baking sheet, spray with butter flavored pam, sprinkle with salt. Bake 375 for 40 min, turn spray again, sprinkle with salt and bake for another 20 min. The salt helps the sugars caramelize.

Serving size 4 oz
Total Calories   71
Total Fat 4.7g
Total Carbs 7.2g
Total Sugar 7g
Total Protein 0.1g

Mashed Sweet Potato

Serves 6
2 lb. of Yams or Sweet Potatoes
2 tablespoons of Extra Virgin Olive Oil
1 tablespoon chopped fresh Rosemary
1 tablespoon chopped Garlic
pinch of Garlic Salt

Clean and perforate yam or sweet potato. Peel off skin, cube and boil to preferred tenderness. Place skinless sweet potato in a bowl, add extra virgin olive oil, chopped rosemary, garlic, sprinkle garlic salt. Mash together with handheld mixer and serve.

Serving size 4 oz
Total Calories   88
Total Fat 2.4g
Total Carbs 17.1g
Total Sugar 3.5g
Total Protein 1g

Sweet Potato Fries

Serves 6
3 large sweet potatoes
Drizzle of olive oil
pinch of salt and pepper

Cut sweet potato in half if it is very large. Then cut it into 3/4 slices. Then into 3/4 strips. Place on baking pan, drizzle with olive oil and sprinkle salt and pepper. Bake at 450* for 15 min, flip and bake for another 10 min.

Serving size 4 oz
Total Calories 80
Total Fat 2.3g
Total Carbs 14g
Total Sugar 6.5g
Total Protein 1g

Sweet Basil Dressing

Serves 10-12
Basil- 3 bunches chopped fresh
1 tablespoon honey
2 teaspoons lemon juice
1/4 cup extra virgin olive oil
1/2 cup seasoned rice wine vinegar
1 tablespoon Fage 0% plain greek yogurt
1/2 cup Water

Blend ingredients together. Add 1-2 Tablespoons to your favorite salad.

Serving size 1 Tablespoon
Total Calories   71
Total Fat 4.7g
Total Carbs 7.2g
Total Protein 0.1g
Total Sugar 7g

Eat it. Lift it. Love it. No Excuses!

Asian Coleslaw

Serves 8-10
Slaw
4 cups shredded cabbage purple or green
2 cups shredded carrots
2 red bell peppers
2 cups cooked edamame
3 stalks green onions finely chopped
1 cup peanuts
1/2 cup chopped cilantro

Dressing
1 tablespoons sweet chili sauce
1 tablespoon honey
1/4cup extra virgin coconut oil
1/4 cup apple cider vinegar
2 tbsp Tamari or Gluten free soy sauce
1 teaspoon roasted sesame seed oil
1 tablespoon peanut butter (natural no sugar   added)
1 tablespoon minced ginger
1 tablespoon minced garlic

Slaw
Combine all slaw ingredients in a large salad bowl.

Dressing
Combine all dressing ingredients in a medium bowl. Stir until coconut oil and peanut butter are smooth and dissolved. add the dressing to the slaw. Toss and allow to sit in refrigerator for about 10-15 minutes so that veggies have time to absorb the flavor. Serve cold.

Serving size 1 cup
Total Calories 251
Total Fat 17.8g
Total Carbs 13.3g
Total Protein 9g
Total Sugar 6.7g

Oven Roasted Vegetable Medley

Serves 4
2 Parsnips
4 Kale Stalks
1 Medium Fennel Bulb
1 Tablespoon Extra Virgin Olive Oil
Fresh Ground Pepper

Preheat oven to 375*. Chop vegetables and place on cookie sheet or any oven roasting pan available. Drizzle with Extra Virgin Olive Oil and sprinkle with pepper. Roast for about 30-45 min or until desired tenderness is reached.

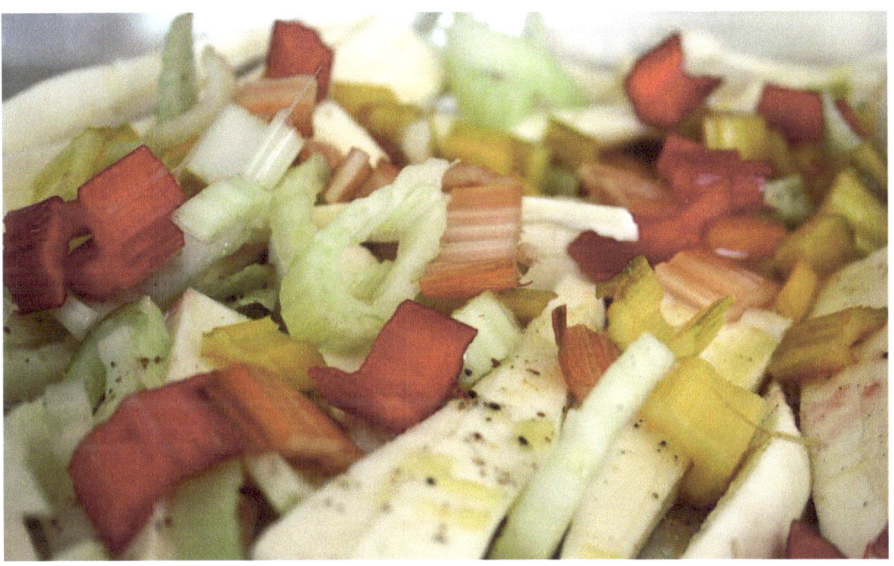

Serving size 1/4 of Mixture
Total Calories 95
Total Fat 3.9g
Total Carbs 15.2g
Total Protein 1.6g
Total Sugar 3.2g

Eat it. Lift it. Love it. No Excuses!

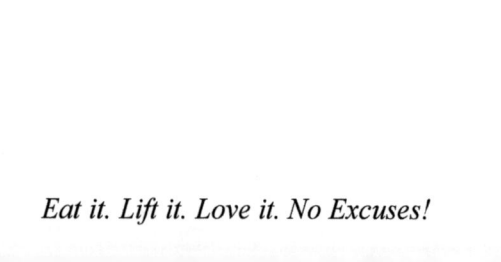

Eat it. Lift it. Love it. No Excuses!

Entrees

Teryaki Protein Plate
Turkey Burger
3 Bean Turkey Chili
Blue Cheese Turkey Muffins
Sloppy Joe's
Thai Chicken and Mushroom Soup
Gluten/Dairy Free Mac and Cheese
Shrimp and Chicken Stir-fry
Chicken Parmigiana
Enchiladas
Easy Shredded Chicken

Eat it. Lift it. Love it. No Excuses!

Chicken Teriyaki

Serves 4
16 oz Chicken Breast
1/2 Cup Organic Brown Rice (Cooked)
2 Tablespoons Teryaki Sauce
1 Cup Chopped Broccoli
1 Cup Baby Carrots (Cooked)
1 Can Organic Black Beans (Drained and Rinsed)
1/8 Cup Diced Onion
1/8 Cup Diced Garlic
1 Tablespoon Sesame Seed Oil

In large skillet sauté onion and garlic with sesame oil over medium heat. Add Chicken when onion starts to turn brown. Sauté until chicken is no longer pink. Add all remaining ingredients and combine until evenly mixed and heated. Serve Immediately.

Serving size 1/4 of Prepared Mixture
Total Calories 266
Total Fat 5.4 g
Total Carbs 7.2 g
Total Protein 26.1g
Total Sugar 4.4g

Turkey Burgers

Serves 6
1 lb. Ground Turkey Lean or Extra Lean
1 whole egg
1 1/2 tablespoons dry Meat Loaf Mix of choice
1/2 cup Gluten Free   Rolled Oats
2 tablespoons Sweet Baby Rays Original BBQ sauce

Mix all ingredients in a medium bowl. Form six equal sized burgers and grill until no longer pink in the center.

Serving size 1 Burger
Total Calories 168
Total Fat 6.7 g
Total Carbs 10 g
Total Protein 13.5 g
Total Sugar 4.5g

Eat it. Lift it. Love it. No Excuses!

3 Bean Turkey Chili

Serves 8

1 lb. Ground Turkey Lean or Extra Lean
1 15oz can Kidney Beans
1 15oz can Garbanzo Beans
1 15oz can Black Beans
1 cup cooked Brown Rice
2 15oz can Tomato Sauce (no sugar added)
2 tablespoons Sweet Baby Rays Original BBQ sauce
2 tablespoons crushed garlic
3/4 Medium Yellow Onion
1/2 tablespoon Tapatio

Brown Turkey in Frying pan. In Large Saucepan, add all other ingredients, add turkey once fully cooked. Simmer for 30min to 1 hour. If cooking for an evening meal it is recommended to exclude Brown Rice in order to lower carbohydrate consumption.

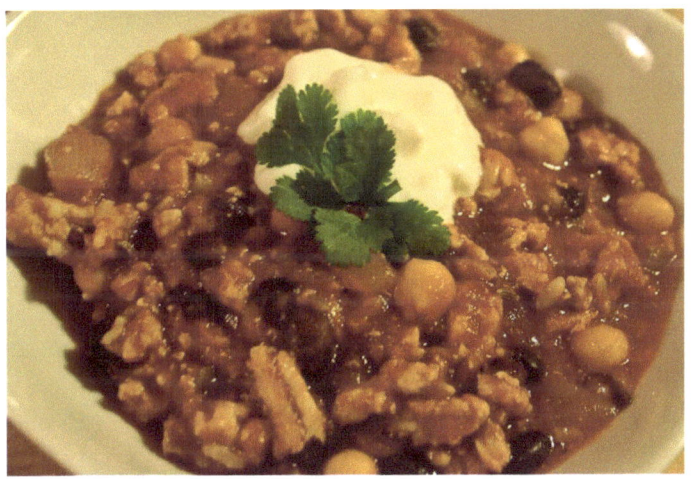

Serving size 1/8 of mixture
    Total Calories 353
    Total Fat 5.7 g
    Total Carbs 44g
    Total Protein 22.4g
    Total Sugar 8.4g

Blue Cheese Turkey Muffins

Serves 10
1 lb. Ground Turkey Lean or Extra Lean
1 whole egg
1 Tablespoon Red Barron Spice
1/2 cup Italian Gluten Free Breadcrumbs
2 tablespoons Ketchup
1/2 cup low fat Blue Cheese

Mix all ingredients in a medium bowl. Form 3oz balls and place in muffin pan. Bake 350 for 23 min. of until fully cooked.

Serving size 2 Muffin
Total Calories 259
Total Fat 8g
Total Carbs 8.9g
Total Protein 34.2g
Total Sugar 2g

Sloppy Joe's

Serves 8
1 lb. Ground Turkey Lean or Extra Lean
1 whole egg
2 Tbsp Sweet Baby Ray's Original BBQ sauce
1 cup Carrots, Shredded
3 medium Zucchini, Shredded
1/2 pack Simply Organic Sloppy Joe Seasoning
1 Onion, Chopped

In Large Skillet, sauté onion, egg and ground turkey until thoroughly cooked. Add carrots and zucchini, cook for 3 min. Add BBQ sauce and seasoning to mixture until well combined. Serve immediately. Adults on the program may enjoy mixture on its own or on 1/2 gluten free multi grain bread or bun.

Serving size 1/8 of mixture
Total Calories 121.7
Total Fat 1.6g
Total Carbs 8.6g
Total Protein 18g
Total Sugar 4.9g

Eat it. Lift it. Love it. No Excuses!

Thai Chicken and Mushroom Soup

Serves 5
2 Chicken Breast thinly sliced
1/2 container Low Sodium Chicken Broth
2 Cans Light Coconut Milk
3 cloves garlic diced
2 tablespoon grated ginger
2 tablespoon lemon grass
1 lime for zest
1 can bamboo shoots drained
1 1/2 tablespoon fish sauce
2 cup Shitake mushrooms sliced
2 carrots shredded
1/4 cup fresh cilantro leaves
1 Serrano pepper, seeds removed, diced
1 medium shallot thinly sliced
1 lime wedged for serving

Combine chicken broth, garlic, ginger, lemon grass, lime zest, fish sauce into a medium sauce pan and bring to a simmer. Simmer for approximately 3 minutes then add mushroom, bamboo shoots, and carrots, simmer for 3 more   minutes. Add chicken and coconut milk and simmer, stirring until chicken is cooked, about 3 more minutes. Serve with cilantro, shallots, lime wedges and Serrano peppers as garnish.

Serving size 1 bowl
Total Calories 268
Total Fat 13g
Total Carbs 12g
Total Protein 23g
Total Sugar 0.3g

Gluten/Dairy Free Mac and Cheese

Serves 10

1 box Quinoa Organic Gluten Free Pasta Elbows
1/4 cup Gluten Free Italian Breadcrumbs
2 cups Raw Cashews
2 tablespoons Tahini Sauce
2 teaspoons lemon juice
1 cup Silk Original Almond Milk
1 teaspoon Extra Virgin Olive Oil
1 teaspoon Garlic Salt
1 teaspoon ground black pepper
1 Pack Turkey Bacon, cooked and chopped
1/2 tablespoon Fennel Seasoning

After soaking cashews for 2 hours at minimum, place in food processor with tahini sauce, lemon juice, almond milk, olive oil, garlic salt and black pepper. Mix in food processor until a   creamy consistency is reached. Cook Quinoa Pasta as directed on package. Drain and add cashew cheese mixture. Mix gently until well combined.   Add turkey bacon to mix. Place mixture in ramekin dishes and preheat oven to 450. Place a thin layer of breadcrumbs on top of mac and cheese m i x and place in oven. Bake only until breadcrumbs turn slightly brown. Remove and serve immediately.

Serving size 1 Ramekin
Total Calories 290
Total Fat 12.7 g
Total Carbs 29.2g
Total Protein 12.1g
Total Sugar 4g

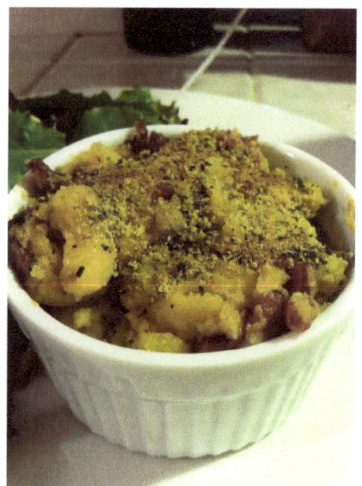

Eat it. Lift it. Love it. No Excuses!

Shrimp and Chicken Stir-fry

Serves 6
2 -16 oz packages of shrimp
1 whole rotisserie chicken
1 cup edamame
2 package sugar snap peas
1 cup shredded carrots
1 can bamboo shoots
1 can water chestnuts sliced
1 cup mung beans sprouts
1/2 cup chicken broth low sodium
3 tablespoons apple cider vinegar
2 tablespoons grated ginger root
3 tablespoons gluten free Tamari sauce

In large skillet or wok over medium high heat, stir fry edamame, carrots, bamboo shoots, water chestnuts, mung bean sprouts and ginger root for 3 minutes. Add all remaining ingredients until well combined and heated. Serve over brown rice or on it own.

Serving size 1/6 of mixture
Total Calories 376
Total Fat 7.9g
Total Carbs 19.6g
Total Protein 44.3g
Total Sugar 8g

Chicken Parmigiana

Serves 5
5 chicken breast
1/2 cup Gluten Free Marinara sauce
3/4 cup Gluten free panko bread crumbs
2 tablespoons Italian Seasoning
1/4 cup Parmesan Cheese-grated
1/4 cup Low Fat Part Skim Mozzarella Cheese
2 tablespoons Extra Virgin Olive oil

Preheat oven for 450*. Lightly spray a large baking sheet with cooking spray. Combine panko breadcrumbs, italian seasoning and parmesan cheese in bowl. Lightly brush extra virgin olive oil onto chicken breast, then dip into the crumb mix. Place on baking dish and repeat for remaining 4 chicken breast. Lightly spray the top of chicken breast, and bake 10 minutes. Flip breast and bake for another 10 minutes. Remove chicken from oven, place two tablespoons of marinara sauce on top of chicken and 1 tablespoon mozzarella cheese on top of marinara. Return to oven and bake for another 5 minutes or until cheese is melted. Serve immediately.

Serving size 4oz Chicken Breast
Total Calories 292
Total Fat 10.4 g
Total Carbs 18.4g
Total Protein 31.6g
Total Sugar 3.2g

Chicken Enchiladas

Serves 6
Chicken
1/2 batch of Easy Shredded Chicken or 1 whole rotisserie chicken shredded without skin.
8 oz Fage 0% Greek Yogurt
1 lime juiced
1/4 cup cilantro
1/2 tablespoon gluten free taco seasoning
Sauce
1 16oz can of tomato sauce sugar free
1 tbsp olive oil
1/2 onion diced
4 garlic cloves diced
1 tbsp Mrs Dash southwest chipotle seasoning
3/4 cup low sodium chicken broth
1 can diced green chilies
12 Corn Tortillas
1 cup shredded low fat Mexican cheese

Preheat oven for 350 degrees. In medium sauce pan, add olive oil, onion, garlic, green chillies and Mrs Dash Chipotle spices. Sauté for 5 minutes. Add tomato sauce, chicken broth and let simmer for 20 minutes. Combine shredded chicken, fage, lime juice, cilantro and taco seasoning in medium bowl.

Spray 13x9in baking dish with non-stick cooking spray. Fill each tortilla with 1/3 cup chicken mixture. Roll it up and place in baking dish seam side down. Top with Sauce and cheese. Cover and bake for 20-25 minutes until cheese is completely melted and starting to brown. Top with scallions and fage greek yogurt.

Serving size two enchilada
Total Calories 274
Total Fat 8.7g
Total Carbs 25.2g
Total Protein 24.5g
Total Sugar 7.9g

Easy Shredded Chicken

Serves 6
3 large chicken breast 10-12 oz each
1 container Organic Low Sodium Chicken Stock

In crockpot on high. Add Chicken breast and cover with chicken stock. Cook for 4 hours. Drain out juices and shred chicken. Great for tacos, salads and enchiladas.

Serving size 1/6 of mixture
Total Calories 169
Total Fat 5.6g
Total Carbs 0.7g
Total Protein 30.1g
Total Sugar 0g

Healthy Desserts

Cinnamon Apples and Cottage Cheese
Pumpkin Dessert Blend
Peanut Butter Cookies

Eat it. Lift it. Love it. No Excuses!

Cinnamon Apple Cottage Cheese

Serves 1
1 Medium Fuji Apple cubed
1 Teaspoon Cinnamon
1/2 cup Low Fat Cottage Cheese

Place cubed chunks of apple in small bowl. Add Cinnamon. Mix well. Top with cottage cheese.

Serving size 1
Total Calories 160
Total Fat 0g
Total Carbs 27g
Total Protein 15 g
Total Sugar 20g

Pumpkin Swirl

Serves 1
1/2 Cup Low Fat Cottage Cheese
1/4 Pumpkin Puree
1 tablespoon Honey
2 teaspoons Pumpkin Pie Seasoning
2 tablespoons Almond Milk

Combine all ingredients into a blender and blend until smooth texture. Refrigerate for 20 min and serve.

Serving size 1
Total Calories 160
Total Fat 0g
Total Carbs 27g
Total Protein 15 g
Total Sugar 20g

Peanut Butter Cookies

Serves 12
1 cup All Natural Peanut Butter
1/2 cup Stevia
1/2 cup Unsweetened Cocoa Powder
2 egg whites
1 tsp baking soda
Pinch of salt

Mix and roll into 12 equal balls, place on greased cooking pan. Press down with fork. Bake at 325 for 13 min.

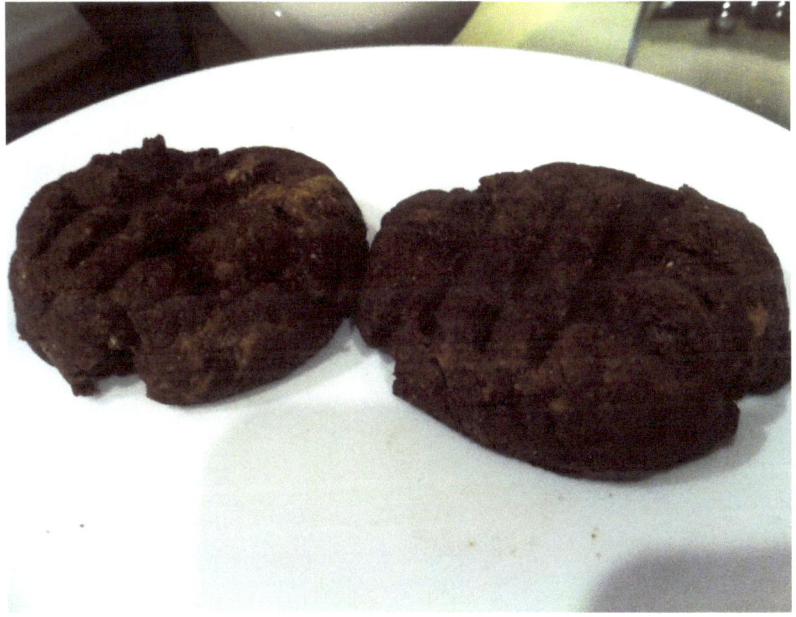

Serving Size 2 cookies
Total Calories 122
Total Fat 8.9g
Total Carbs 4.3g
Total Protein 6g
Total Sugar 1g

Eat it. Lift it. Love it. No Excuses!

Eat it. Lift it. Love it. No Excuses!

Holiday Recipes

Too Tart Cranberry Sauce
Crustless Pumpkin Pie
Green Beans
Herb Roasted Turkey

Real Cranberry Sauce

Serves 14
1 package of whole cranberry
1 medium orange
1 medium apple
1/2 tablespoon orange zest
1/4 cup stevia
1 cup currants

Place whole cranberries, sugar and orange juice in blender. Blend to desired consistency. Place in bowl, stir in currants, and garnish with zest of an orange.

Serving size ~1/4 cup
Total Calories 50
Total Fat 0g
Total Carbs 12.9g
Total Protein 0.5g
Total Sugar 11g

Crustless Pumpkin Pie

Serves 8
5 egg whites
1- 15 oz can pure pumpkin
1/3 cup stevia
3 tbsp rice flour
1 cup dry milk
1/2 tsp nutmeg
1/2 tsp cinnamon
1/2 tsp pumpkin pie seasoning

Combine all ingredients in a large bowl. Spray 9 in pan with butter cooking spray. Pour batter into pan. Bake at 350* for 45-55 minutes or until a toothpick comes out clean. Refrigerate for 30 min to one hour prior to serving.

Serving size 1 slice-pie cut into 8 pieces
Total Calories 155
Total Fat 0.3 g
Total Carbs 24.4 g
Total Protein 15g
Total Sugar 20.3g

Eat it. Lift it. Love it. No Excuses!

Green Beans

Serves 6
1/4 cup pine nuts
2 lb. of green beans
2.5 tsp extra virgin olive oil
1 sliced of smoked ham cut into small pieces
4 cloves of garlic
1/2 yellow onion finely chopped

In large pot, bring water to a boil. Add beans and cook until they are crisp-tender. Drain and set aside. Heat extra virgin olive oil in skillet over medium heat. Add onion, garlic, and ham. Sauté until ham is browned and garlic and onions are fully cooked. Add green beans cook until beans are slightly browned. Stir in pine nuts and serve.

Serving size 1cup
Total Calories 152
Total Fat 10.3 g
Total Carbs 9.4 g
Total Protein 9.3g
Total Sugar 0.8 g

Herb Roasted Turkey

Serves 12
1 18 lb Turkey
1 cup low sodium chicken stock
2 lemons
2.5 tsp extra virgin olive oil
1/8 tsp pepper
4 sprigs of rosemary
2 sprigs of Thyme
4 cloves of garlic
/2 yellow onion finely chopped

Preheat oven for 375 degrees. Prepare Turkey as instructed. Wash and remove giblets and parts. Pat dry and place in roasting pan. Chop lemons into 4 pieces and place inside turkey along with 3 rosemary, 1 thyme, garlic and onion. Tie legs of turkey together on outside of turkey rub olive oil onto skin. Finely chop remaining rosemary and thyme and mix with pepper. Rub herbs on to skin. Pour chicken stock in the bottom of the pan. Place in oven and bake for 2 hours uncovered or until turkey skin has browned, basting every 30 minutes. Once turkey is browned, baste again and place lid on roasting pot or cover with tinfoil. Continue to cook until internal temp reaches 180 degrees, approximately 4 1/4 hours. When done let sit for 20 minutes before serving.

Serving size 4 oz of white turkey meat
Total Calories 180
Total Fat 8 g
Total Carbs 0 g
Total Protein 24g
Total Sugar 0g

Serving size 4 oz of dark turkey meat
Total Calories 262
Total Fat 10g
Total Carbs 0g
Total Protein 40g
Total Sugar 0g

Eat it. Lift it. Love it. No Excuses!

HERES YOUR PROOF! IT WORKS!

This is my first progress photo! This is what you can do in as little as 3 months on The Program. Lose weight, lose inches, gain muscle and self confidence! I am my own walking billboard.

- Ashley Ross, Age 27, Creator of The Program

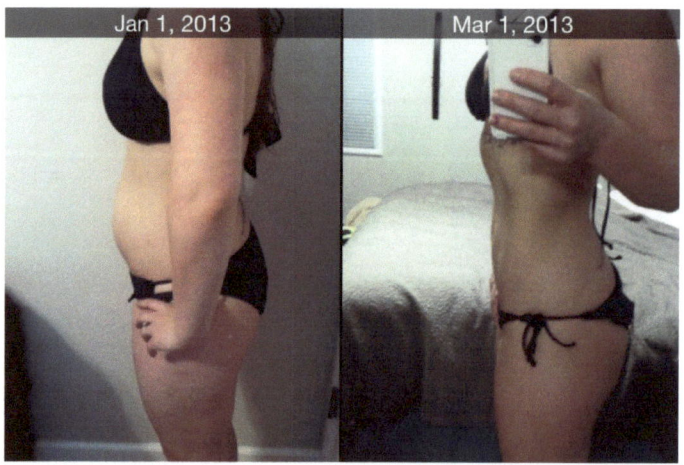

-Stephen Ross, Age 36, Creator of The Program

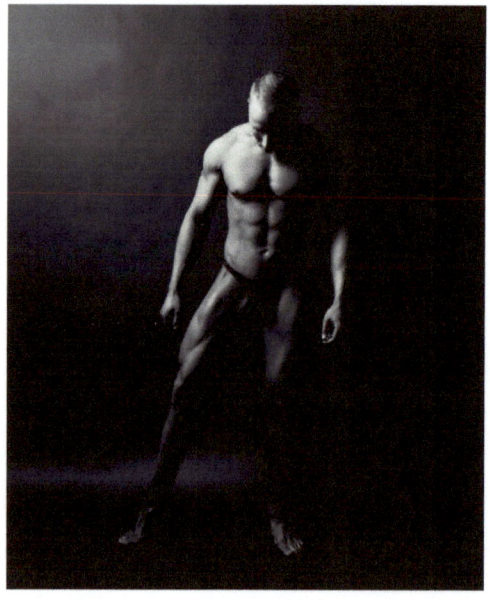

Eat it. Lift it. Love it. No Excuses!

www.ingramcontent.com/pod-product-compliance
Lightning Source LLC
Chambersburg PA
CBHW040326010626
45792CB00024B/2148